Making-use of

CIALIS

(TA-DA-LA-FIL) Tablets

The Full-blown Fast Acting Cialis (Tadalafil)
Guide to Get Hard and Stay Hard with
Long-Lasting Erection for Her Full-blown
Screaming Blue Sex Climax

Dr. Robert Bratt

Table of Contents

Chapter 1

PROLOGUE TO MALE LIFE STRUCTURES

1.1 An Outline of the Male Regenerative Framework

The male regenerative framework is a wonder of natural designing, unpredictably intended with the end goal of sexual multiplication. Involving an organization of organs and designs, this framework guarantees the creation, development, and conveyance of sperm — the infinitesimal specialists of treatment.

Testes:

Situated inside the scrotum, the testicles are the essential male conceptive organs liable for sperm creation (spermatogenesis) and chemical emission. These little, oval-molded organs house seminiferous tubules, where sperm cells are delivered, and Leydig cells, which discharge testosterone.

Epididymis:

Connected to every gonad, the epididymis fills in as a stockpiling and development site for sperm. During its excursion through the epididymis, sperm go through fundamental changes, acquiring the capacity to treat an egg.

Vas Deferens:

This solid cylinder transports developed sperm from the epididymis to the urethra during discharge. The vas deferens assumes a significant part in the impetus of sperm towards their final location.

Prostate Organ and Original Vesicles:

These adornment organs contribute liquids to semen, feeding and upgrading the portability of sperm. The prostate organ encompasses the urethra and is liable for creating a smooth liquid, while the original vesicles contribute a fructose-rich liquid that gives energy to sperm.

1.2 Grasping the Design and Capability of the Penis

The penis, an image of male virility and sexuality, is a complicated organ with particular designs and works.

Shaft:

The shaft of the penis comprises of three sections of erectile tissue — two corpora cavernosa and one corpus spongiosum. These tissues load up with blood during excitement, prompting an erection.

Glans:

The glans, or top of the penis, is wealthy in sensitive spots, making it profoundly touchy. It assumes a urgent part in sexual joy and feeling.

Erectile Tissues:

The corpora cavernosa and corpus spongiosum are liable for the mechanics of an erection. When engorged with blood, these tissues make the immovability essential for sex.

1.3 The Job of Chemicals in Sexual Wellbeing

Chemicals go about as synthetic couriers, arranging different cycles inside the male regenerative framework.

Testosterone:

Created essentially in the testicles, testosterone impacts the advancement of male conceptive organs, sperm creation, and the sign of auxiliary sexual qualities. It is likewise basic to keeping up with moxie and generally speaking sexual prosperity.

Gonadotropins:

Chemicals, for example, luteinizing chemical (LH) and follicle-invigorating chemical (FSH) control testosterone creation and sperm development.

Key Action items:

The male conceptive framework includes an organized exertion of organs and designs.

The penis has a modern life structures vital for sexual capability.

Chemicals, especially testosterone, assume a critical part in keeping up with sexual wellbeing.

Chapter 2:

HOW ERECTIONS OCCUR

2.1 Investigating the Physiological Course of Erection

Erection, a key part of male sexual capability, is a wonder of perplexing physiological cycles. Understanding how this peculiarity happens is pivotal for valuing the intricacy and excellence of male sexual reaction.

Sexual Excitement:

The excursion towards an erection commonly starts with sexual excitement, set off by tactile upgrades, contemplations, or feelings. This starts an outpouring of occasions in the body, making way for the physiological reaction.

Arrival of Synapses:

Upon sexual excitement, the mind cues the arrival of synapses, like nitric oxide (NO), which assume a critical part in the unwinding of smooth muscle cells in the penis.

Unwinding of Smooth Muscle:

The arrival of nitric oxide prompts the unwinding of smooth muscle cells inside the erectile tissues of the penis. This unwinding permits blood to stream into the veins of the penis, engorging the erectile chambers.

Blood Inflow:

As the smooth muscle unwinds, blood stream to the penis increments fundamentally. The two corpora cavernosa and the corpus spongiosum, made out of wipe like erectile tissues, load up with blood, making the penis become unbending and erect.

Catching of Blood:

To keep up with the erection, veins that typically channel blood away from the penis choke, catching blood inside the erectile tissues. This supported blood stream is fundamental for the upkeep of a firm erection.

2.2 The Interaction of Veins, Nerves, and Chemicals

The course of erection includes a modern transaction of veins, nerves, and chemicals, featuring the intricacy of male sexual physiology.

Veins:

Corridors conveying oxygenated blood to the penis widen, working with expanded blood stream. At the same time, veins tighten to forestall the fast surge of blood, keeping up with the engorgement of erectile tissues.

Nerves:

The sensory system assumes a vital part in sending signals between the mind and the penis. Tangible improvements and sexual considerations start nerve driving forces that lead to the arrival of synapses, adding to the unwinding of smooth muscle.

Hormones:

Hormonal equilibrium, especially including testosterone, is fundamental for the inception and upkeep of the physiological cycles related with erection. Disturbances in hormonal levels can affect sexual capability.

2.3 Normal Elements Influencing Erectile Capability

A few elements can impact erectile capability, either emphatically or adversely. Understanding these elements is fundamental for perceiving likely difficulties and looking for suitable mediations.

Mental Variables:

Stress, nervousness, wretchedness, and other mental variables can essentially influence sexual excitement and erection. The brain body association is vital in keeping up with sound sexual capability.

Way of life Elements:

Undesirable way of life decisions, including horrible eating routine, absence of activity, and substance misuse, can add to conditions like stoutness, diabetes, and cardiovascular issues, which may adversely influence erectile capability.

Ailments:

Certain ailments, like diabetes, hypertension, and neurological issues, can affect the veins and nerves engaged with the erection interaction.

Medications:

A few drugs, including specific antidepressants, antihypertensives, and narcotics, may have secondary effects that influence sexual capability.

Key Action items:

Erections are a complex physiological reaction to sexual excitement.

The transaction of veins, nerves, and chemicals coordinates the interaction.

Mental, way of life, clinical, and prescription related elements can impact erectile capability.

Chapter 3:

FACTORS INFLUENCING SEXUAL WELLBEING

3.1 Talking about Way of life Variables Influencing Sexual Execution

Sexual wellbeing is impacted by a horde of way of life factors that stretch out past the actual parts of the body. This part digs into the more extensive setting of what everyday decisions and propensities can altogether mean for sexual execution.

Inactive Way of life:

An absence of actual work is related with different medical problems, including corpulence and cardiovascular issues, which can think twice about stream to the private parts and add to erectile brokenness.

Smoking and Substance Misuse:

Tobacco and sporting medication use have been connected to lessened sexual execution. These substances can influence blood course and may add to conditions influencing sexual wellbeing.

Liquor Utilization:

While moderate liquor utilization is for the most part viewed as adequate, unnecessary drinking can prompt sexual brokenness. Liquor goes about as a depressant, influencing both physiological and mental parts of sexual capability.

3.2 The Job of Pressure, Diet, and Actual work in Sexual Wellbeing

Stress and Uneasiness:

Elevated degrees of stress and tension can upset the fragile equilibrium of chemicals associated with sexual capability. Persistent pressure might add to conditions like erectile brokenness and diminished drive.

Diet and Sustenance:

A fair and nutritious eating routine is fundamental for in general wellbeing, including sexual wellbeing. Certain supplements, for example, zinc and omega-3 unsaturated fats, assume a part in hormonal guideline and blood stream, impacting sexual capability.

Active work:

Customary activity has been related with worked on sexual capability. Actual work improves cardiovascular wellbeing, advances appropriate blood flow, and adds to generally speaking prosperity, which are all indispensable to sexual wellbeing.

3.3 Normal Misinterpretations About Male Sexual Capability

Age and Sexual Execution:

In opposition to mainstream thinking, progress in years alone doesn't decide sexual ability. While maturing can achieve changes in sexual capability, keeping a sound way of life can relieve many age-related factors influencing sexual wellbeing.

Size and Execution:

A typical misinterpretation spins around the connection between's penis size and sexual fulfillment. Actually, profound association, correspondence, and common assent assume more huge parts in sexual satisfaction.

Recurrence of Erections:

Another confusion includes the conviction that incessant erections are demonstrative of sexual wellbeing. The recurrence of erections can fluctuate among people and may not be guaranteed to associate with generally speaking sexual capability.

Key Action items:

Way of life factors, including actual work and substance use, influence sexual wellbeing.

Stress, diet, and exercise assume urgent parts in keeping a solid sexual capability.

Normal confusions about age, size, and recurrence of erections can impact impression of sexual wellbeing.

Chapter 4:

PROLOGUE TO CIALIS

4.1 Comprehension Cialis as a Phosphodiesterase Type 5 (PDE5) Inhibitor

Cialis, likewise known by its conventional name Tadalafil, is a drug delegated a phosphodiesterase type 5 (PDE5) inhibitor. This part gives a top to bottom investigation of how Cialis capabilities to address erectile brokenness.

PDE5 Hindrance:

Cialis works by repressing the activity of the catalyst PDE5, which is answerable for separating cyclic guanosine monophosphate (cGMP). By hindering PDE5, Cialis expands cGMP levels, advancing smooth muscle unwinding and upgrading blood stream to the penis during sexual feeling.

Length of Activity:

One striking component of Cialis is its delayed term of activity contrasted with other PDE5 inhibitors. This lengthy window, frequently as long as a day and a half, has procured Cialis the epithet "the end of the week pill," giving more noteworthy adaptability to sexual immediacy.

4.2 How Cialis Contrasts from Other Erectile Brokenness Meds

Cialis is important for a class of meds intended to address erectile brokenness, however it has remarkable qualities that recognize it from different medications inside a similar class.

Length of Activity:

Dissimilar to some other PDE5 inhibitors, for example, Viagra and Levitra, Cialis has a more drawn out span of activity. This lengthy window permits people to take part in sexual action without the time imperatives related with different drugs.

Beginning of Activity:

While the beginning of activity might differ among people, Cialis is known for its moderately quick beginning, with impacts becoming recognizable in something like 30 minutes to an hour after ingestion.

Day to day versus On-Request Use:

Cialis offers the choice for everyday use at lower dosages, offering ceaseless help for erectile capability. This recognizes it from different meds that are regularly taken dependent upon the situation.

4.3 Proper Utilization, Measurement, and Likely Aftereffects

Proper Utilization:

Cialis is endorsed for the treatment of erectile brokenness in men. Understanding when and how to utilize Cialis is essential for expanding its advantages.

Measurements Rules:

Doses might change in view of individual necessities and wellbeing contemplations. This segment gives direction on choosing the fitting Cialis dose and the significance of counseling medical services experts for customized suggestions.

Expected Incidental effects:

While for the most part very much endured, Cialis, similar to any drug, might be related with specific secondary effects. This part frames normal aftereffects and stresses the significance of looking for clinical consideration in the event that unfriendly responses happen.

Key Action items:

Cialis is a PDE5 inhibitor, improving erectile capability by expanding cGMP levels.

Exceptional qualities, including a lengthy term of activity, recognize Cialis from other erectile brokenness prescriptions.

Fitting use, measurement contemplations, and potential incidental effects ought to be talked about with medical care experts.

Chapter 5:

INSTRUMENT OF ACTIVITY

5.1 Investigating How Cialis Upgrades Erectile Capability

Understanding the system by which Cialis works reveals insight into its adequacy in tending to erectile brokenness. This section digs into the many-sided processes through which Cialis upgrades erectile capability.

PDE5 Hindrance:

Cialis goes about as a strong inhibitor of phosphodiesterase type 5 (PDE5), a significant compound in the guideline of smooth muscle tone in the penis.

By repressing PDE5, Cialis delays the presence of cyclic guanosine monophosphate (cGMP), an optional courier that works with smooth muscle unwinding.

Smooth Muscle Unwinding:

Raised degrees of cGMP lead to the unwinding of smooth muscle cells inside the erectile tissues of the penis.

This unwinding considers expanded blood stream into the enormous assemblages of the penis, bringing about engorgement and the advancement of an erection.

5.2 The Effect of PDE5 Hindrance on Blood Stream to the Penis

Blood vessel Expansion:

PDE5 inhibitors, including Cialis, advance the expansion of corridors providing blood to the penis.

This blood vessel widening increments blood stream, guaranteeing a sufficient inventory of oxygen and supplements to the erectile tissues.

Venous Tightening:

All the while, PDE5 restraint prompts the choking of veins that normally channel blood away from the penis.

This choking keeps up with the engorgement of the erectile tissues, supporting the erection all through sexual movement.

5.3 Length of Activity and Timing Contemplations

Expanded Span:

One of the distinctive elements of Cialis is its lengthy span of activity, enduring as long as a day and a half at times.

This drawn out window gives people expanded adaptability, considering suddenness in sexual movement.

Beginning of Activity:

While individual reactions might shift, Cialis normally displays a generally quick beginning of activity, with impacts becoming observable in something like 30 minutes to an hour after ingestion.

Timing Contemplations:

To enhance the advantages of Cialis, people are educated to consider the timing regarding organization, guaranteeing that the prescription is taken inside the suggested time period before expected sexual action.

Key Action items:

Cialis upgrades erectile capability by repressing PDE5 and expanding cGMP levels.

PDE5 hindrance advances blood vessel expansion and venous narrowing, upgrading blood stream to the penis.

Cialis separates itself with its drawn out term of activity and somewhat quick beginning, giving adaptability in timing.

Chapter 6:

Advantages and Contemplations

6.1 Talking about the Advantages of Cialis Past Erectile Brokenness

Cialis, famous for its adequacy in treating erectile brokenness, offers extra advantages that stretch out past the domain of sexual capability. This section investigates the more extensive benefits related with the utilization of Cialis.

1. Treatment of Pneumonic Blood vessel Hypertension (PAH):

Cialis is endorsed for the treatment of pneumonic blood vessel hypertension, a condition described by raised pulse in the pneumonic veins.

By loosening up the smooth muscle in aspiratory veins, Cialis further develops practice limit in people with PAH.

2. Improvement in Exercise Resistance:

A few examinations recommend that Cialis might upgrade practice resilience in people with different cardiovascular circumstances.

The vasodilatory impacts of Cialis add to expanded blood stream, possibly helping with the improvement of generally speaking cardiovascular capability.

6.2 Possible Purposes in the Treatment of Harmless Prostatic Hyperplasia (BPH)

1. Alleviation of Lower Urinary Plot Side effects (LUTS):

Cialis has been endorsed for the treatment of lower urinary parcel side effects related with harmless prostatic hyperplasia (BPH).

By loosening up smooth muscle in the prostate and bladder, Cialis mitigates side effects, for example, trouble peeing and continuous pee.

2. Mix Treatment:

At times, medical services suppliers might recommend Cialis in blend with different prescriptions for the administration of BPH, giving a far reaching way to deal with side effect help.

6.3 Distinguishing Circumstances Where Cialis May Not Be Reasonable

1. Prior Ailments:

People with specific ailments, like extreme liver or kidney infection, may require measurements changes or cautious observing while utilizing Cialis.

2. Contraindications:

Cialis is contraindicated in people utilizing nitrate drugs because of the gamble of a possibly serious drop in pulse.

Alert is educated in those with a set of experiences regarding cardiovascular sickness, as sexual action itself might represent a specific degree of hazard.

3. Associations with Different Meds:

Expected associations among Cialis and different drugs ought to be thought of. It is fundamental to illuminate medical services suppliers regarding all prescriptions, including over-the-counter and home grown supplements.

Key Action items:

Cialis expands its advantages past erectile brokenness to conditions, for example, aspiratory blood vessel hypertension and lower urinary lot side effects related with BPH.

Its utilization in BPH plans to mitigate side effects by loosening up smooth muscle in the prostate and bladder.

Cautious thought is required in circumstances where Cialis may not be appropriate, including previous ailments and contraindications with specific prescriptions.

Chapter 7:

WAY OF LIFE CHANGES FOR SEXUAL PROSPERITY

7.1 Executing an All-encompassing Way to deal with Sexual Wellbeing

A comprehensive way to deal with sexual prosperity includes sustaining the actual parts of the body as well as the psychological, profound, and social features of one's life. This section investigates the interconnectedness of different way of life factors that add to generally sexual wellbeing.

1. Profound and Mental Prosperity:

Stress, nervousness, and sorrow can influence sexual longing and execution. Participating in exercises that advance close to home prosperity, for example, care practices and treatment, can decidedly impact sexual wellbeing.

2. Correspondence and Relationship Elements:

Transparent correspondence with an accomplice encourages a strong and grasping climate, vital for keeping a solid sexual relationship.

7.2 Dietary Proposals and Nourishing Help

1. Adjusted Diet:

A nutritious and adjusted diet is essential for generally wellbeing, including sexual prosperity. Supplement rich food varieties add to cardiovascular wellbeing, chemical guideline, and energy levels.

2. Explicit Supplements for Sexual Wellbeing:

Certain supplements, like zinc, omega-3 unsaturated fats, and cancer prevention agents, assume parts in supporting regenerative wellbeing and hormonal equilibrium.

3. Hydration:

Keeping up with satisfactory hydration is fundamental for by and large wellbeing and can emphatically influence sexual capability.

7.3 The Job of Customary Activity and Stress The board

1. Cardiovascular Activity:

Ordinary active work, particularly cardiovascular activity, upgrades blood flow, adding to worked on erectile capability.

2. Strength Preparing:

Strength preparing activities can advance generally speaking wellness, adding to expanded endurance and imperativeness.

3. Stress The board Strategies:

Persistent pressure can adversely influence sexual wellbeing. Stress the board procedures, like reflection, profound breathing, and yoga, can assist with reducing pressure and work on generally prosperity.

4. Quality Rest:

Sufficient and quality rest is fundamental for hormonal equilibrium, energy levels, and by and large wellbeing, all of which add to sexual prosperity.

7.4 Tracking down the Right Equilibrium

1. Control in Propensities:

Balance in liquor utilization and aversion of tobacco and sporting medications add to in general wellbeing and sexual prosperity.

2. Looking for Proficient Direction:

People confronting difficulties in their sexual wellbeing are urged to look for direction from medical care experts, including sexual wellbeing trained professionals and advisors.

Key Focal points:

A comprehensive way to deal with sexual prosperity considers profound, mental, and social elements.

A decent and nutritious eating routine, alongside unambiguous supplements, upholds generally speaking wellbeing and conceptive capability.

Normal activity, stress the board, and sufficient rest add to upgraded sexual prosperity.

By integrating these way of life changes, people can make an establishment for worked on sexual wellbeing and by and large prosperity. It's memorable's essential that sexual wellbeing is a multi-layered part of one's life, and an exhaustive methodology is much of the time the way to long haul achievement. The ensuing sections will keep on investigating useful contemplations for keeping up with and streamlining sexual wellbeing.

Chapter 8:

FUTURE TURNS OF EVENTS AND END

8.1 Investigating Progressing Exploration in the Field of Sexual Wellbeing

1. Propels in Accuracy Medication:

Continuous examination is making ready for additional customized ways to deal with sexual wellbeing. Accuracy medication might prompt customized medicines in light of a person's hereditary cosmetics, enhancing remedial results.

2. Neurobiological Bits of knowledge:

Headways in neurobiology are disentangling the many-sided associations between the mind and sexual capability. Understanding the brain systems included may open new roads for designated mediations.

3. Hormonal Treatments:

Examination into hormonal treatments keeps, investigating creative ways of regulating hormonal levels and address uneven characters that add to sexual brokenness.

8.2 Expected Headways in Prescriptions and Medicines

1. Novel PDE5 Inhibitors:

The advancement of new phosphodiesterase type 5 (PDE5) inhibitors might offer other options or upgrades over existing prescriptions, giving improved viability and decreased incidental effects.

2. Quality Treatments:

Quality treatments are not too far off, with scientists exploring ways of adjusting qualities related with sexual capability. This notable methodology might offer long haul answers for specific sexual ailments.

3. Integrative Methodologies:

Consolidating pharmacological mediations with psychotherapy, way of life changes, and elective treatments might turn into a standard work on, offering a far reaching and individualized way to deal with sexual prosperity.

8.3 A Closing Synopsis and Support for Looking for Proficient Counsel

1. All encompassing Way to deal with Sexual Wellbeing:

The excursion to ideal sexual wellbeing includes an all encompassing point of view that considers physical, close to home, and social perspectives. Way of life changes, meds, and potential future progressions all assume urgent parts in this excursion.

2. Individualized Care:

Perceiving that every individual's involvement in sexual wellbeing is exceptional, it is foremost to look for proficient guidance. Medical services suppliers, including sexual wellbeing subject matter experts, can offer customized direction in light of a singular's particular necessities and conditions.

3. The Significance of Open Correspondence:

Open correspondence with medical care experts and accomplices is fundamental. Examining concerns, objectives, and treatment choices encourages a cooperative way to deal with accomplishing and keeping up with sexual prosperity.

4. Consolation for a Sound Future:

All in all, this guide has planned to give experiences into the complexities of sexual wellbeing, underscoring the significance of a proactive and all encompassing methodology. By remaining informed, looking for proficient guidance, and embracing continuous progressions, people can explore their sexual wellbeing venture with certainty and positive thinking.

Key Focal points:

Progressing research investigates accuracy medication, neurobiological experiences, and hormonal treatments for sexual wellbeing.

Expected headways in prescriptions incorporate novel PDE5 inhibitors, quality treatments, and integrative methodologies.

An all encompassing methodology, individualized care, open correspondence, and support for looking for proficient exhortation are fundamental for a solid sexual future.

As the field of sexual wellbeing keeps on developing, people are urged to remain informed, take part in open correspondence, and look for proficient direction to guarantee a sound and satisfying sexual life. May this guide act as an important asset on your excursion towards ideal sexual prosperity.

Printed in Great Britain
by Amazon

33010418R00035